For My

Daughter

on the Birth

of Her

First Child

For My Daughter on the Birth of Her First Child

*A Keepsake
Journal
from Mother
to Daughter*

Developed by
BookEnds, LLC

HYPERION
NEW YORK

Book design by Ruth Lee

Library of Congress Cataloging-in-Publication Data

For my daughter on the birth of her first child : a keepsake journal from mother to
  daughter. — 1st ed.
      p. cm.
    ISBN: 0-7868-6682-9
    1. Baby books. 2. Childbirth — Miscellanea. 3. Mothers — Diaries.

HQ779.F668 2001
306.874'3—dc21   00-044967

FIRST EDITION

10   9   8   7   6   5   4   3   2   1

I want you to have this very special book because . . .

....
....
....
....
....
....
....
....
....
....

The relationship between a mother and a daughter is something that no one—outside of another mother and daughter—will ever truly understand. It is one of love, deep friendship, and admiration. At the same time, this relationship is made up of two people who are often too much alike, too entirely different, too proud, and too embarrassed of each other all at once.

Your mother is someone who is always there for you. She makes you chicken soup when you are sick, holds your hand when you are scared, and dries your tears when you are sad. She is the only person you can trust to always tell the truth . . . even if you don't want to hear it. And there is no one like a mother with whom to share your greatest happinesses. She will always be there, watching your life story unfold, watching you change from a dependent little girl into a powerful, mature woman. And as the major rites of passage come upon you in life, she will support you, love you, and witness your changes.

The birth of a first child is a momentous occasion in life. It is a time of great hope, great fear, and intense love. And for mother and daughter it is a time of enormous change and an opportunity for a unique intimacy. A daughter is about to become a mother herself, and mother and daughter will now understand each other on an entirely new level. You will probably feel closer to each other than you have ever felt before. Suddenly you are equals: caretakers, supporters, and nurturers of the highest order.

Not only is this a time of joy and hope, but it can also be a time of struggle and disagreement. It is a time to record your feelings, your hopes, your fears, and your dreams, and to lay the groundwork for the path of the future.

For My

Daughter

on the Birth

of Her

First Child

Two of a Kind

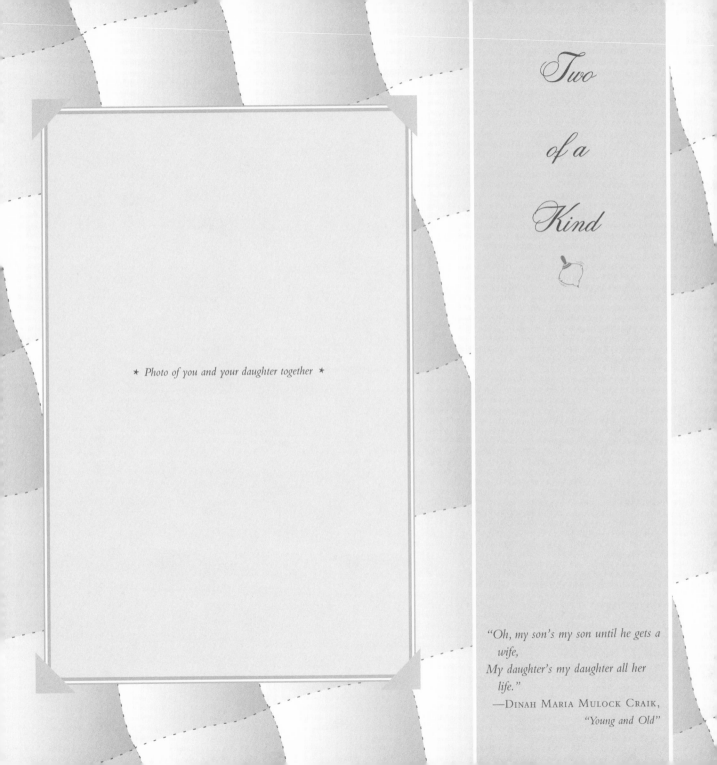

★ *Photo of you and your daughter together* ★

"Oh, my son's my son until he gets a wife,
My daughter's my daughter all her life."
—DINAH MARIA MULOCK CRAIK,
"Young and Old"

My Treasure

I love you so much because . . .

I think our relationship is special because . . .

"Wrinkles are hereditary. Parents get
them from their children."
—DORIS DAY

A Mother's Work Is Never Done

Being your mother has been . . .

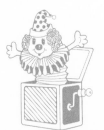

I think you are like me in the following ways:

....
....
....
....
....
....
....
....
....
....

I think you are like your father in the following ways:

....
....
....
....
....
....
....
....
....
....
....

Separated

at Birth

I hope your baby has your . . .

When I think of you as a little girl, I always think of . . .

7

Sweet

Surrender

"We dress them in the presumptions of
the world. They are the bright small
face of hope. They are the last belief
we have, the belief in making them
believe."

—E. L. DOCTOROW

You made me laugh when you . . .

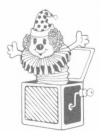

You made me cry when you . . .

I'll never forget the time we . . .

....
....
....
....
....
....
....
....
....
....
....
....
....
....
....
....
....
....
....
....
....
....
....
....

"The soul is healed by being with children."

—FYODOR DOSTOYEVSKI

I have never been so proud of you as when . . .

Like

Mother,

Like

Daughter

You'll make a wonderful mother because . . .

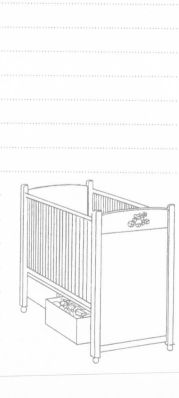

Grandma

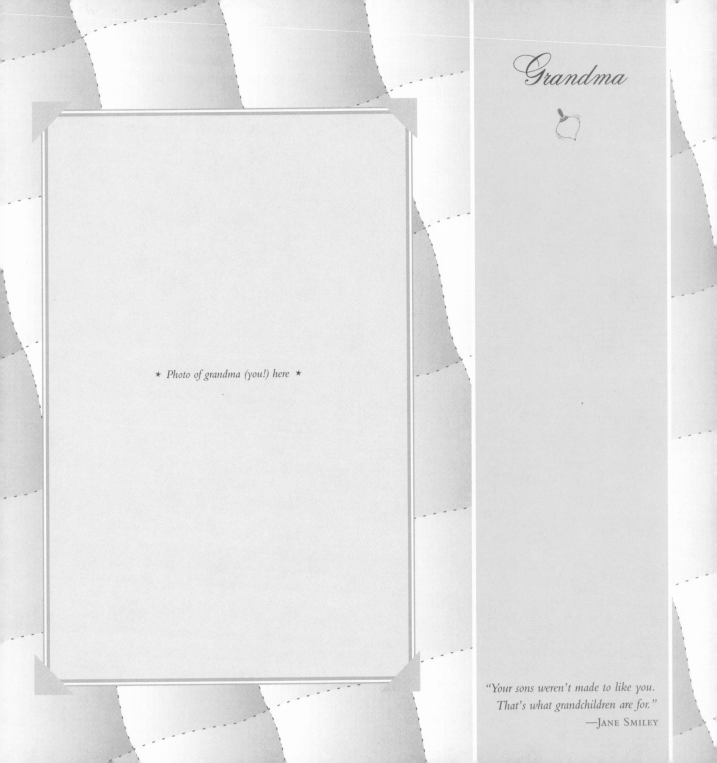

★ *Photo of grandma (you!) here* ★

"Your sons weren't made to like you.
That's what grandchildren are for."
—Jane Smiley

It's a Grandma!

When you first told me you were going to have a baby, I thought . . .

....

....

....

....

....

....

....

....

....

I felt . . .

....

....

....

....

....

....

....

....

....

The first words out of my mouth were . . .

"Elephants and grandchildren never forget."

—ANDY ROONEY

Hello, Borneo!!

I immediately told . . .

I am most excited because . . .

Pink

or

Blue?

I hope you have a girl because . . .

....

....

....

....

....

....

....

....

....

I hope you have a boy because . . .

....

....

....

....

....

....

....

....

"As is the mother, so is the daughter."
—THE BOOK OF THE PROPHET
EZEKIAL, 16:44

I would like to be the kind of grandmother who . . .

Memory Lane

Photo of you and your husband as a young couple, prebaby

"No one like one's mother and father
ever lived."
—ROBERT TRAILL SPENCE LOWELL,
"Returning"

I first found out I was pregnant with you when . . .

Surprise!

My first thought was . . .

"The first duty to children is to make them happy. If you have not made them so, you have wronged them. No other good they may get can make up for that."

—CHARLES BUXTON

I hoped you were a girl because . . .

Sugar

and

Spice

The girl names I chose were:

"A girl is innocence playing in the mud . . ."

—ALAN BECK

I hoped you might be a boy because . . .

The boy names I chose were:

....

....

....

....

....

....

....

....

....

....

....

....

....

....

....

....

....

....

....

....

....

....

....

....

....

"The name we give to something shapes our attitude toward it."
—KATHERINE PATERSON

I found out you were a girl when . . .

....

....

....

....

....

....

....

....

....

I thought . . .

....

....

....

....

....

....

....

....

....

....

....

A Babe in Pink

When I told your dad I was pregnant, he said this:

The first thing I bought for you when I was pregnant was . . .

Did

Somebody

Say

Shopping?

I pictured you as . . .

The Pregnancy

Photo of pregnant you

"*Familiarity breeds contempt—and children.*"

—Mark Twain

What I liked most about being pregnant was . . .

What I liked least was . . .

Gummy Bears with Ketchup, Please!

I craved . . .

. . . .

. . . .

. . . .

. . . .

. . . .

. . . .

. . . .

. . . .

. . . .

. . . .

. . . .

. . . .

. . . .

. . . .

. . . .

. . . .

. . . .

. . . .

I gained . . .

....
....
....
....
....
....
....
....
....
....
....
....
....
....
....
....
....
....
....
....
....
....
....

Are You

Sure It's

Not Twins?

I had the following symptoms:

....
....
....
....
....
....
....
....
....
....
....
....
....
....
....
....
....
....
....
....
....
....
....

I had the following dreams:

....
....
....
....
....
....
....
....
....
....
....
....
....
....
....
....
....
....
....
....
....
....

Stranger in the Mirror

My body changed in strange ways. What I remember most was:

My breasts . . .

....

....

....

My belly . . .

....

....

....

My thighs . . .

....

....

....

My skin . . .

....

....

....

My arms . . .

....

....

....

My feet . . .

....

....

....

My back . . .

....

....

....

My bottom . . .

....

....

....

My womb . . .

....

....

....

My face . . .

....

....

....

When I lay in bed at night, I hoped for . . .

....

....

....

....

....

....

....

....

....

....

I was frightened of . . .

....

....

....

....

....

....

....

....

....

....

....

"To fear is one thing. To let fear grab
you by the tail and swing you
around is another."
—KATHERINE PATERSON

Things I wish I had known . . .

....

....

....

....

....

....

....

....

Things I wish I hadn't known . . .

....

....

....

....

....

....

....

....

Twinkle,

Twinkle,

Little Star

"The child must know that he is a miracle, that since the beginning of the world there hasn't been, and until the end of the world there will not be, another child like him."
—PABLO CASALS

A Family Affair

* Photo of entire family *

"*Always be nice to your children because they are the ones who will choose your rest home.*"
—PHYLLIS DILLER

Your father and I agreed on . . .

Harmony

Your father and I disagreed on . . .

Your father wanted a girl because . . .

Your father wanted a boy because . . .

46

Your father was funny when he . . .

....

....

....

....

....

....

....

....

....

....

....

....

....

....

....

....

....

....

....

....

....

....

Laughter,

the Best

Medicine

"I want to have children while my parents are still young enough to take care of them."
—RITA RUDNER

My mother's advice to me was . . .

My father's advice to me was . . .

Be Yourself

My advice to you is . . .

"During much of my life I was anxious to be what someone else wanted me to be. Now I have given up that struggle. I am what I am."

—ELIZABETH COATSWORTH

When we told your grandparents I was pregnant with you, they said . . .

....

....

....

....

....

....

....

....

....

....

....

When I told your grandmothers you were pregnant, they said . . .

....

....

....

....

....

....

....

....

....

....

....

"Kids are wonderful, but I like mine barbecued."

—BOB HOPE

The Delivery

★ *Photo of you and your newborn daughter* ★

"Every child is born a genius."
—R. BUCKMINSTER FULLER

When my water broke, I . . .

....

....

....

....

....

I went into labor at . . .

....

....

....

....

....

....

I was in labor for . . .

....

....

....

....

....

....

Here Comes the Flood

"It is somehow reassuring to discover that the word travel *is derived from* travail, *denoting the pains of childbirth."*

—JESSICA MITFORD

This is what my labor was like:

....
....
....
....
....
....
....
....
....
....
....
....
....
....
....
....
....
....
....
....
....
....

I liked my doctor because . . .

I didn't like my doctor because . . .

What I packed in my suitcase to go to the hospital:

What I thought about on the drive to the hospital:

....
....
....
....
....
....
....
....
....
....
....
....
....
....
....
....
....
....
....
....
....
....
....
....
....

I wished I had brought the following with me to the hospital:

I was scared about . . .

What I would do differently:

What I'd do all over again:

What they say is true about . . .

....
....
....
....
....
....
....
....
....
....
....
....
....
....
....
....
....
....
....
....
....
....
....
....
....
....
....

It Doesn't

Hurt

at All

What they say isn't true about . . .

The pain was . . .

....
....
....
....
....
....
....
....
....
....
....
....
....
....
....
....
....
....
....
....
....
....

*"There was no reality to pain when
it left one, though while it held
one fast all other realities failed."*
—RACHEL FIELD

Please, Sir, May I Have Some More?

My advice about an epidural is . . .

Questions I'd ask my doctor today:

....

....

....

....

....

....

....

....

....

....

....

....

....

....

....

....

....

....

....

....

....

....

....

....

....

Yes,

Chocolate

Pudding.

I'd make sure the doctor knew exactly how I felt about . . .

....
....
....
....
....
....
....
....
....
....
....
....
....
....
....
....
....
....
....
....
....
....

Your dad was/was not there during the birth because . . .

I did/did not want him there because . . .

....
....
....
....
....
....
....
....
....
....
....
....
....
....
....
....
....
....
....
....
....
....
....
....

The funniest thing I said in labor was . . .

....

....

....

....

....

....

....

....

....

....

....

....

....

....

....

....

....

....

....

If You

Ever Come

Near Me

Again . . .

The funniest thing your dad did during the delivery was . . .

When the nurse put you in my arms, I thought . . .

The Most Beautiful Girl in the World

Your father looked at you and he said . . .

....

....

....

....

....

....

....

....

....

....

....

....

....

....

....

....

....

....

It took me this long to lose the pregnancy weight:

....
....
....
....
....
....
....
....
....
....
....
....
....
....
....
....
....
....
....
....
....
....
....

Aftercare

These were some of the aftereffects of being pregnant and giving birth that I experienced:

....

....

....

....

....

....

....

....

....

....

....

....

....

....

....

....

....

....

....

....

....

....

....

I recommend taking care of yourself in these ways:

Baby Girl

* Photo of your daughter as a toddler *

"There's only one pretty child in the
world, and every mother has it."

—PROVERB

You weighed:

....
....
....
....
....
....
....
....
....
....
....

Your were _____ inches long.

....
....
....
....
....
....
....
....
....
....
....
....

Perfection

The first time I nursed you . . .

....

....

....

....

....

....

....

....

....

....

I nursed you for this long:

....

....

....

....

....

....

....

....

....

....

....

What I think about nursing:

"Adam and Eve had many
advantages, but the principle one
was that they escaped teething."
—MARK TWAIN

Bliss

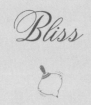

The most indescribably wonderful thing about those first few days was . . .

You didn't sleep through the night until . . .

....

....

....

....

....

You ate solid food at . . .

....

....

....

....

....

I used the following tricks to get you to eat:

....

....

....

....

....

Your favorite foods were . . .

....

....

....

....

....

"If this was adulthood, the only improvement she could detect in her situation was that she could now eat dessert without eating her vegetables."

—LISA ALTHER,
Kinflicks

You would never eat . . .

....
....
....
....
....
....
....
....
....
....

You were potty trained at . . .

....
....
....
....
....
....
....
....
....
....

You first spoke at . . .

....
....
....
....
....
....
....

Your first words were . . .

....
....
....
....
....
....
....

You took your first steps at . . .

....
....
....
....
....
....
....

Not the Lipstick!

You always got into . . .

....

....

....

....

....

....

....

....

....

....

....

....

....

....

....

....

....

....

....

....

*"Parents who are afraid to put their
foot down usually have children who
step on their toes."*

—CHINESE PROVERB

I thought you were the greatest thing in the world because . . .

....

....

....

....

....

....

....

....

....

....

....

....

....

....

....

....

....

....

....

....

....

*"God could not be everywhere and
therefore he created mothers."*
—JEWISH PROVERB

Utter

Perfection

I thought you were different because . . .

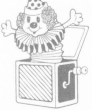

I worried that . . .

You made me laugh when you . . .

Motherhood made me feel . . .

"To understand your parents' love
you must raise children yourself."
—CHINESE PROVERB

I was terrified that . . .

I felt irrevocably changed both inside and outside in these ways:

Personal Favorites

Your favorite story was . . .

....
....
....
....
....
....
....
....
....
....
....
....
....
....
....
....
....
....
....
....
....

"Who is the fairest one of all?"
—Snow White

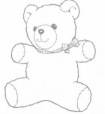

Your favorite toy was . . .

Your favorite cartoon was . . .

Your favorite nursery rhyme was . . .

"Mary, Mary, quite contrary . . ."

Your favorite Disney character was . . .

I couldn't take this away from you without major repercussions:

....

....

....

....

....

....

....

....

....

....

....

....

....

....

....

....

....

....

....

....

....

....

Like

Candy

from a

Baby . . .

Your funniest feature as a baby was . . .

My advice to you about TV is . . .

My advice to you about your pediatrician is . . .

....

....

....

....

....

....

....

....

....

....

....

....

....

....

....

....

....

....

....

....

....

....

....

The best advice I can give you on motherhood is . . .

....

....

....

....

....

....

....

....

....

....

....

....

....

....

....

....

....

....

....

....

Love,

Love,

Love

"The best way to keep children home is to make the home atmosphere pleasant—and let the air out of the tires."

—DOROTHY PARKER

Take care of yourself—don't neglect *your needs*. Make time for . . .

I think you will make a terrific mother because . . .

"A mother is not a person to lean
on, but a person to make leaning
unnecessary."
—DOROTHY CANFIELD FISHER

Wish List

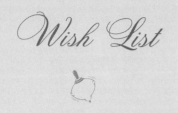

I would like to be the kind of grandmother who . . .

....
....
....
....
....
....
....
....
....
....
....
....
....
....
....
....
....
....
....
....
....
....
....
....

These are my dreams for you as a mother . . .

"A dream is a wish your heart makes . . ."
—*Cinderella*

Family

Traditions

★ *Photo of entire family here* ★

Special family traditions and where they came from:

....

....

....

....

....

....

....

....

....

....

....

....

....

....

....

....

....

....

....

....

....

....

....

....

....

....

....

Holiday

Traditions

Family

Stories

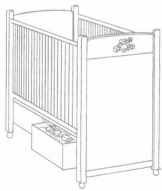

Family Facts . . .

GRANDPARENTS

Names	DOB	Death	Height/Weight	Health

PARENTS

Names	DOB	Death	Height/Weight	Health

Outstanding family characteristics:

....

....

....

....

....

....

....

....

....

....

....

....

....

....

....

....

....

....

....

....

....

....

....

....

....

Family

Recipes

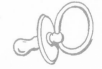

Family Tree